The Smart & Easy Guide To Migraine & Headache Relief: Diagnosis, Treatments, Lifestyle, Resources & Cultural Help For Migraine Headaches & Chronic Pain in Men, Women, Kids, Students & Employees

Sara Lowery

Legal Stuff

COPYRIGHT

DISCLAIMER

THIS BOOK IS NOT DESIGNED TO, AND DOES NOT, PROVIDE MEDICAL ADVICE. ALL CONTENT ("CONTENT"), INCLUDING TEXT, GRAPHICS, IMAGES AND INFORMATION AVAILABLE IN OR THROUGH THIS BOOK ARE FOR GENERAL INFORMATIONAL PURPOSES ONLY.

THE CONTENT IS NOT INTENDED TO BE A SUBSTITUTE FOR PROFESSIONAL MEDICAL ADVICE, DIAGNOSIS OR TREATMENT. NEVER DISREGARD PROFESSIONAL MEDICAL ADVICE, OR DELAY IN SEEKING IT, BECAUSE OF SOMETHING YOU HAVE READ ON THIS BOOK. NEVER RELY ON INFORMATION ON THIS BOOK IN PLACE OF SEEKING PROFESSIONAL MEDICAL ADVICE.

THE AUTHOR, PUBLISHER AND ALL AFFILIATED PARTIES ARE NOT RESPONSIBLE OR LIABLE FOR ANY ADVICE, COURSE OF TREATMENT, DIAGNOSIS OR ANY OTHER INFORMATION, SERVICES OR PRODUCTS THAT YOU OBTAIN THROUGH THIS SITE. YOU ARE ENCOURAGED TO CONFER WITH YOUR DOCTOR WITH REGARD TO INFORMATION CONTAINED IN OR THROUGH THIS BOOK. AFTER READING THIS BOOK, YOU ARE ENCOURAGED TO REVIEW THE INFORMATION CAREFULLY WITH YOUR PROFESSIONAL HEALTHCARE PROVIDER.

Table of Contents

HISTORY OF MIGRAINES (DIAGNOSIS & TREATMENT)

A migraine is a circumstance in which a person suffers from an extreme pain in the brain, which is caused by different, sometimes contradicting factors. While the term "Migraine" is a newly coined term in the modern age, the idea of an intense headache dates back to the early ages of Man, to the point that it can be regarded as one of the oldest diseases identified.

Due to this, methods of diagnosing and treating this condition have varied through the centuries.

Ancient Methods of Treatment

Ancient Egyptians believed that migraines are preternatural in nature, and so they used to cure them by rubbing a friend fish directly into the affected area. This method is purely superficial in nature, and no medical basis exists as to why this kind of treatment works, if any.

Later on, the Egyptians developed a different method of treatment, still using superficial methods, by tying a clay crocodile to the patient's head using a strip of linen. On the linen, names of different Egyptian deities that were believed to cure any diseases were written. This method, while still superficial in nature, does possess some basis in modern medicine due to the fact that migraines can be cured by compressing the scalp and collapsing the blood vessels, which forms the basis of massage being one of the effective methods of migraine treatment.

All of these Egyptian treatment methods are incorporated in the Ebers Papyrus, named so after George Ebers, who obtained it. In this ancient document, various methods of treatment employed by the ancient Egyptians are contained, including those for the treatment of shooting pains in the brain, the exact definition of migraines.

During the middle ages, the cure for migraine consisted mostly of a mixture of opium and vinegar, which is then applied to the skull. The vinegar's purpose is supposed to open up the pores of the brain so that the opium may pass through, thereby curing it. Withal, as opium is now in the list of banned medicines of today, the procedure eventually faded.

Famous People Who Have Defined Landmarks in Migraine Diagnosis & Treatment

Plato is considered one of the world's greatest philosophers of all time. However, his opinion about migraines might be considered wrong, especially to modern people. According to Plato, migraines are only the result of people paying too much attention to their body instead of their brains. Which means the migraine condition is just "in their heads", a purely mental condition. While some people might agree about this philosophy of Plato, most of today's people will not.

In 460 BC, Hippocrates, the well-known "Father of Medicine", already established the symptoms of migraines well ahead of his time. He described the condition as a shining light that is usually seen in one eye and accompanied by severe pain that starts right about the temples and slowly works its way around, eventually spreading over to the entirety of the head and neck. Hippocrates also was one of the first people to relate headaches to intensive exercise, and even severe sexual intercourse. He also noted that migraines could also result from vapors formed from the acids in the abdomen that can also work their way up to the head region, and noted that treatment from this can be achieved by simply vomiting.

Hua T'o, a Chinese surgeon who lived in the second century, was credited for the invention of anesthetic drugs to cure different kinds of conditions, migraines included. He's also one of the first doctors to use acupuncture needles to cure migraines, though this can be subjected to debate, as acupuncture has been part of Chinese medicine for a long time. One particularly famous case during Hua T'o's medicine career was when he cured suffering from pain between his eyes because of a tumor. After he carved the tumor out of the patient, a canary suddenly flew out, and the man not only was cured of his pain, but he also lived.

Hildegard of Bingen was a medieval nun and mystic who is known for experiencing various kinds of visions at an early age. Her visions eventually inspired her to write several books related to medicine, health and also natural remedies. Due to her written accounts, as well as the illustrations that she drew herself, many people now believed that her visions are likely the result of migraine auras, which is mainly attributed to the vividness and clarity of her artworks, and her descriptions are clear and well detailed. It is then that she became one of the first migraine-inspired artists, eventually establishing a following.

As technology advances and many new discoveries happen, it can be safe to say that the treatment for migraines will also evolve as well. Soon enough, all our curing methods of today may become obsolete and abandoned in favor of newer, more advanced methods in the future.

FAMOUS MIGRAINE PATIENTS

You may believe that you're just one of the very few people who suffer from a migraine when it attacks. Well the truth is, migraines are actually a very common condition, as much as a common cold. Moreover, you might be surprised that, not only is it incredibly commonplace, but several famous people are also known to have suffered this condition, and some of them have even developed famous works of art because of it.

Here's an exhaustive list of the famous people who have had migraines in the past, classified by their profession:

• Famous Writers – Many well-known writers in the past were actually migraine sufferers, who actually used this condition to their advantage to write their famous works. One of the best examples is Lewis Carroll (Charles Lutwidge Dodgson) who is believed that his famous work, "Alice in Wonderland" is actually inspired from one of his migraine attacks.

Other famous people who made some literary works based on their migraine conditions include Virginia Woolf and Miguel de Cervantes. One of Emily Dickinson's written poems is also based on her migraine suffering, describing it as "coffin nails".

• Famous Politicians – Well-known politicians in the past have also been frequent migraine sufferers. The best examples of rulers who suffer from this condition are the infamous Roman dictator Julius Caesar, and the infamous French emperor, Napoleon Bonaparte, who almost succeeded in conquering most parts of the world.

In America, the famous President and author of the Declaration of Independence, Thomas Jefferson, also experienced several migraine attacks, particularly during the time he was writing it. While in the American Civil War, the two commanders on the opposing sides of the war, Robert E. Lee (Confederacy Commander) and Ulysses S. Grant (Union Commander), also suffered from this condition.

• Famous Painters – Just like writers, some famous painters also drew their artwork inspiration from their migraine suffering episodes. The legendary Vincent Van Gogh, whose vivid colours and elegant brush strokes are believed to have resulted from the auras he experienced from his migraine attack. Georges Seurat, who created the painting technique called "Pointilism", who used small dots of color to create a large image, were also thought to be experiencing a migraine aura when he got the technique, due to the similarities that it has.

• Famous Celebrities – It is common belief that most, if not all, celebrities also suffer from migraine attacks, and some of them have openly expressed it themselves. Among those who suffered from migraines is the illustrious King of Rock & Roll himself, Elvis Presley.

Other notable celebrities who admitted to have suffered migraine attacks include actress and comedienne Whoopi Goldberg, British Royal Family member Princess Margaret, sister of Queen Elizabeth II, and even Susan Olsen, the actress who is well-known for portraying Cindy Brady of "The Brady Bunch". Janet Jackson even had some of her shows cancelled because of certain migraine attacks.

Several celebrities also tried to manage their migraine attacks through different methods. Marcia Cross (Desperate Housewives) became a spokesperson for the migraine treatment drug, Imitrex. Lisa Kudrow (Friends) used lidocaine as a migraine treatment, while Carly Simon has successfully managed hers via proper diets.

• Famous Athletes – While known as being physically fit, some athletes have also suffered from several migraine episodes during the course of their careers. One of the well-known ones is the famous NBA player Dwayne Wayde, who wears tinted glasses whenever he play to manage them, and Percy Harvin, who actually managed to cure his migraine via proper diet and regular physical therapy. Freddie Ljungberg, a famous Swedish soccer player, even had to be carried off the field once when he suffered a migraine attack mid-game. Almost the same situation happened to Terell Davis, star player of the Denver Broncos who suffered a migraine during the Super Bowl XXXII, forcing him to miss the second quarter. Due to his ample education on this condition, however, Davis was able to continue playing around halftime, and eventually earned himself an MVP award for this. Serena Williams, the tennis player, even went on to become a spokesperson for the "RALLY for Menstrual Migraine" campaign.

• Others – The father of psychoanalysis himself, Sigmund Freud, has also reputed to have suffered migraines during his life. The famous Saint Joan of Arc (Jeanne D'Arc), has also been reputed to have suffered migraines, which explained her reputed visions, according to modern scholars. Friedrich Nietzsche, a famous philosopher, has developed the concept of the "Uberman", a certain master race, though many now also attribute this concept to his migraine episodes. And two of the most famous historical people who have revolutionized our thinking are also migraine patients: Charles Darwin, and Albert Einstein.

MIGRAINE IN CULTURE AND THE ARTS

Migraine is a dangerous kind of headache that no one would wish upon even his or her worst enemy. Nevertheless, no one can deny that this level of pain has inspired some of the most artistic accomplishments. After all, people say that great pain also brings about great art. If we were to talk about migraine inspiring pieces in culture and the arts, that adage may very well be true.

Painters are experts in the process of using their pain as an inspiration for creating pieces that will express their passion. The visual effect of the typical migraine aura has been used for artistic expression in different disciplines, across different medium and across various genres. The first notable depiction of migraine aura involves pieces of a medieval artist who is known to everyone as Hildegard of Bilgen. This artist did not only use migraine aura as inspiration to create astounding pieces, but also researched extensively about the subject.

It seems to be true that artists who are suffering from the many effects of debilitating migraine turn to surrealism to express their feelings and their pain. It is a recorded fact that Georgia de Chirico, a surrealism artist, was a frequent migraine sufferer. Salvador Dali, noted for producing the most visual images that depict visual hallucinations, also related to migraine aura.

There are different websites that show and explain so-called "migraine art" and museums have held exhibitions about this kind of art as well. As a matter of fact, there are migraine art competitions! In these competitions, entries are judges based on how artists have translated and produced compositions that depict migraine-induced visions of their minds to the canvas. Artists are asked to create pieces that will expound on the feelings that are supported by those who are experiencing migraine attacks and migraine headaches.

There are different kinds of artistic pieces that have been inspired by migraines. One of the most famous pieces is the Alice in Wonderland books penned by Lewis Carroll. These books are prime examples of literature that is inspired by migraines and these books are also among the most widely read pieces in the universe! Joan Didion's essay entitled "In Bed" is a strong and dependable account of her frequent battles with this condition. Some people even say that this essay is one of the most honest works that has been written about a debilitating ailment. Also, there's "Lady of Lights" by Karla J. Dorman, which is a clinging recreation of the various visual disturbances that are caused by migraines. Everyone who has received a migraine attack and who has grown frantic over the zigzagging lines and shooting stars that danced in front of these eyes during these painful times will surely appreciate how Dorman described the phenomenon as a circus. "The Remarkable Case of Davidson's Eyes" by H.G. Wells is also believed to be a migraine-inspired piece.

The list of artists who have produced wonderful pieces that are supposed to have been inspired by migraine does not stop there! Among the most famous names in culture and the arts, the following artists are supposed to have created works that are inspired by this kind of severe headache and include the following: Vincent Van Gogh, Georgia O'Keefe, William Blake, Gill Knox, Peggy Hoffman, Angela Butt, Neel Kar, Mark Fitzgerald, Sofia Greene, Molly Bass, and many more.

Naturally, there are also music pieces that are supposed to have been made due to the experience brought about by migraines, despite the fact that listening to music is generally not conducive to treating migraines. After all, people tend to be very sensitive to noise when they are suffering from a migraine attack. Musical compositions that were inspired by this ailment were not necessarily created during the attacks, but were formed together during the days when the migraine sensation is still fresh on the minds of the artists.

Some of the greatest musical icons that are known to have suffered from headaches are Elvis Presley and Gustav Mahler. Jeff Tweedy from a group called "Wilco" is also a well-documented sufferer of this condition.

An example of musical works that were inspired by migraine is "Migraine Induced Madness" by Brad Preston. Sources claim that the artist wrote this piece while he was suffering the symptoms of migraine. Other migraine-inspired and titles pieces from big musical artists include the following: The Coral's "Migraine" from the album Nightfreak and the Sons of Becker, Puddle of Mudd's "Migraine" from the album Abrasive, D.J. Signify's "Migraine" from the album Sleep No More, Trouble Hubble's "Migraine" from the album Broken Airplanes, and many more.

IMPORTANT INFORMATION ABOUT MIGRAINES AND WOMEN

Compared to men, women are more prone to experiencing migraine attacks. As a matter of fact, the rate of frequency of migraine in adult women falls somewhere between 15 to 17 percent, while the rate for men falls somewhere close to five percent. Studies show that estrogen withdrawal is a big factor on why women usually experience migraine when they are menstruating. 25 to 30 percent of women who are in the 30 years and above age bracket experience occasional migraines. Even worse, if these migraine attacks are brought about by their menstrual cycle, the pain and discomfort is said to last much longer than non-menstrual attacks. Menstrual migraine attacks are also much trickier to cure.

60 to 70 percent of women experience menstruation-related migraine attacks. As a matter of fact, 10 to 14 percent of these women only experience this condition when they are menstruating. This kind of attacks falls under the category that is known as "true menstrual migraine". In addition to this kind of migraine, women are also prone to experiencing premenstrual migraines as a part of premenstrual syndrome or PMS. In addition to the depression, bloating, fatigue and irritability brought about by PMS, women also have to deal with extreme headache.

A certain percentage of women who have suffered from pre-menstrual migraine are pleased to discover that their condition improved once they entered the phase of physiological menopause. As a matter of fact, two-thirds of women are said to experience this positive turn of events. Nevertheless, surgical menopause, on the other hand, is said to increase the pain and suffering experienced by two-thirds of documented cases.

Pregnant women are usually spared from experiencing migraine attacks. However, there are instances when women experience severe migraine attacks during the first trimester of the pregnancy, with the symptoms of migraine disappearing during the third month.

EFFECTIVE MENSTRUAL MIGRAINE TREATMENT

Women who are thinking of using drugs in order to treat menstrual migraines should consider using non-steroidal and non-inflammatory medications or NSAIDS. The best and the most effective NSAIDS that effectively treat menstrual migraines are ketopfren (Orudis), naproxen (Naprosyn), fenoprofen calcium (Nalfon), ibuprofen (Advil and Motrin), and nabumetone (Relafen).

To achieve the best results, usage of NSAIDs should begin at least two to three days before the actual menstrual flow. Therapy should also be continued throughout the remaining menstrual period. Some women have been said to experience certain gastrointestinal effects, but these cases are nothing serious.

Taking an NSAID is also effective for women who wish to continue their use of birth control devices. Nevertheless, for these cases, therapy should begin on the 19th day of the cycle and should continue until the second day of the next cycle.

There are also other kinds of treatment that woman can consider in the process of dealing with the pain that is caused by migraine. Taking pain relievers like aspirin, acetaminophen, and ibuprofen is usually an efficient route. Women can also consider using estrogen patches in order to numb the pain caused by migraine. Taking daily doses of magnesium also helps in treating menstrual migraine. In addition to these suggestions, taking vitamin B2 of an herb known as feverfew will also reduce the frequency and severity of migraine headaches.

Women who are thinking about trying any of these recommendations should seek the approval of their doctors prior to doing so. This is because individual people have unique health profiles, physiology, and history that should be considered before accepting any kind of medication.

MIGRAINE INCIDENTS AMONG KIDS

While it is common for adults to have migraines, especially women, there are also possibilities that children will see this kind of headache. Unlike tension headaches, migraines are not brought about by tension or stress. On the other hand, migraines are the consequences of a biochemical process that results from the expansion and the contraction of the blood vessels that are found on the patients' brains. Believe it or not, an estimated number of 5% of children suffer from migraine. Both genders experience migraine during their younger years. However, during puberty, females develop better chances of suffering from this condition than males. This is due to the fact that females develop certain hormones during puberty.

Children who are as young as four years old may be diagnosed with migraine. Nevertheless, it is important to recognize that diagnosing migraine cases in children will lead to a trial and error process. Most of the time, migraines are only pinpointed to be the cause of the headache only after worse conditions have been ruled out. Besides, there is also the need to scrutinize the health history of both parents, both for the neurological and physical aspects. Different kinds of tests need to be implemented before cases of migraine in children are pinpointed.

Most of the time, children who suffer from migraines have inherited the condition from their parents. If your family has a clear history of migraine, then it is highly advised that you observe whether your child is showing the signs and symptoms of this ailment or not. If your child is prone to experiencing motion sickness, then there is a big possibility that he or she will develop migraines later in life. In addition to motion sickness, kids who are prone to suffer from migraines when they grow up may also experience disturbances in their sleeping patterns.

For minors, the throbbing pain that is one of the many symptoms of migraine is enough to confuse them from enjoying everyday activities. For this reason, make sure that you tell your child's teacher about their condition. This way, they will be able to implement the necessary treatment if and when your child experiences a migraine attack at school.

As with migraines suffered by adults, migraine auras may or may not be seen by children who suffer from migraine. Auras refer to the visual experiences that normally come with migraine attacks, like flashing lights and dancing stars. However, unlike migraine attacks that are experienced by adults, attacks experienced by the younger ones do not last longer than three or four hours. The downside is that attacks can have worse manifestations despite being shorter on durations, like loss of consciousness, loss of ability to speak, and loss of sensation all over the body.

For children, migraine is often referred to as the "Alice in Wonderland" Syndrome. This occurrence usually involves hallucinations, misses in depth and size perceptions, and distortion of images and patterns. As a matter of fact, there is a hypothesis that the author of Alice in Wonderland himself, Lewis Carroll, was a frequent sufferer of migraine. According to this hypothesis, the hallucinations that he experienced during migraine attacks influenced the direction that his books followed.

Medications are necessary components of migraine treatment for children. Most of the time, taking acetaminophen and other anti-inflammatory medications like ibuprofen do wonders for children who are experiencing migraine attacks. If over the counter drugs do not provide your child the relief that he needs, it may be time to take him to a doctor and to get a prescription. There are drugs that are used to effectively relieve the pain and discomfort caused by this kind of headache, but you will need to bring a note from your doctor or physician before you can get your hands on them.

In addition to learning the necessary MEDs, children who are suffering from frequent migraines are advised to keep "headache diaries" that will allow them to keep track of the different things that trigger their headache. These diaries may also be used to keep track of the different means through which they were able to alleviate the pain that they felt. Most of the time, sleeping, breathing, biofeedback techniques, and acupuncture help in relieving migraine among children.

There are also different kinds of non-drug therapies that you can consider for your child, like stress management and meditation. Make sure that your child also gets all the nutrients and vitamins that they need, in addition to getting enough exercise regularly.

If you have an inkling that your child is suffering from migraine attacks, then make sure that you arrange a date with a doctor as soon as possible. Try to keep track of the following information as well to make the diagnosis easier for you and your child:

- Number of headaches experienced per week

- Intensity of headaches

- Exact location of headaches

- Duration of the headaches

- Foods, drinks, and activities that triggered the headaches

WHAT TO DO IN CASE OF STUDENT MIGRAINES

According to the records of the American Council for Headache Education, school nurses deal with at least 10 cases of headache every month. A large portion of these complaints turns out to be migraine headaches. If you are under the impression that migraine only happens to adults, then take a look through the accompanying figures.

• 38% to 83% of children aged 7 to 15 experience recurring headaches

• 1% to 37% of children ages 3 to 6 experience recurring headaches

• 1.2% to 11% of children experience migraine headaches

Most people fail to realize how much of a problem headaches can be for children. It is a fact that children who are younger than 18 years old experience headaches numerous times every year, from tension headaches, to cluster headaches, to migraines. The occurrence of headaches among females becomes more frequent during puberty, with more teenage girls experiencing migraine headaches than teenage boys. This is mainly due to the fact that estrogen is developing in the female body during this stage in life, especially during the onset of menstruation.

There are certain signs that you should watch out for in order to determine whether migraine is beginning to be too much to handle for your child. If your child seems to be complaining a lot about his or her headache, then there is a good chance that he or she is suffering from migraine attacks. These headaches usually happen in school, where there can be too much brain stimuli.

When a student complains about a potential migraine attack, take note of the context in which the complaint is made. Be wary of students who fake migraine attacks just so they can skip the next lesson. When a student starts complaining, try to ascertain the presence of telltale symptoms that characterize a migraine attack.

Make sure that you also take note of the assertions made by the student who is suffering from a headache. If he or she claims that he is experiencing the worst headache that he or she has ever felt, then the situation may be worse than it appears. Try to determine if the student holds a temperature or if there is stiffness in the neck. If these signs are present, then migraine may be the cause of the problem.

Teachers need to take it upon themselves to pick out whether students are experiencing migraine attacks or not. Headaches and migraine will make going to school a torturing ordeal. In addition to hindering the student from performing his best, the different symptoms of migraine attacks will also bring the fun out of taking part in academic and extracurricular activities.

Even worse, extreme headaches may be signs of worse weather, like a tumor or depression. Teachers need to take it upon themselves to investigate further, for they are usually less threatening for the children, as compared to the parents. Children are usually more comfortable talking about their headache history to their tutors.

There are also various things that teachers can do in order to help students cope with migraine headaches. While these tricks will not necessarily treat the pain, employing these techniques will make it easier for the students to deal with migraine in a school environment.

• Make students get their own water bottles to school. This will make it easier for them to get their dose of fluids for the day.

• Students should be encouraged to get 8 to 10 hours of sleep every night. Teachers should seek to encourage good reading habits that will allow the students to cope with their course work without having to stay up too late.

• Students should also learn good eating habits. For students who are prone to having migraine headaches, foods like cheeses, caffeine, chocolates, and meats should be consumed sparingly.

• Stress and strain are the biggest migraine triggers. If the teacher notices that students are already taking on too much, the teacher should take it upon himself to make school work easier for the family.

• Even the smallest complaints should be taken seriously. If a student complains of a headache, he or she should be transported to the school nurse immediately.

DEALING WITH MIGRAINE AND PREGNANCY

Regardless of how hard we try to avoid it, there will come a point is our lives that migraine attacks just happens without explanation sometimes. It is unfortunate that sometimes it happens in very peculiar situations. That being the case, it's only a matter of chance when migraine strikes a pregnant woman. Don't be naïve and think that it cannot happen in the 9 months of pregnancy, because the law of averages says otherwise.

Our normal treatment for migraine is the problem. Normally, when a migraine attack happens, a person simply takes medication. Admittedly, he must do so with care because every pill does come with a side effect; but when we're talking about a pregnant woman in the same scenario, the decision whether to consume medication or not becomes a lot tougher. In addition, we do not have a clue what most headache medication might bring to a pregnant woman. It is due to this reason that women who wish to be pregnant need to taper off their usual headache medication in advance. Of course, not all cases can consider tapering off their medication because of the amount of pain they experience with their migraine. In such cases, too many factors and risks have to be considered that it is highly advised that you make these decisions with your doctor. Under the guidance of a doctor, a person is more educated during times when a difficult decision has to be made. It is well known that there are medications for migraine that have led to birth defects, while others have shown more promising – less risky results like beta blockers and tricyclics. It is important to observe though that if your relief for migraine is in the form of an injectable, like Imitrex, then you'll have to ask your doctor for a better – less harmful type of medication suited for pregnant women.

The reason why women are advised to consult their doctor before they even begin conception is that birth defects often happens in the first trimester. When there is no consolation, what usually happens is that women with migraine do not think about the implications that might happen to their baby if they persist in their migraine medication. Thus, before a woman becomes pregnant, she must confer with her doctor first because there are a lot of things that pregnant women do that may increase the likelihood of headaches to occur. During pregnancy, hormone imbalance is usually the culprit for eating more food than usual, sleeping later at nights, mood swings, etc.... all of which are common triggers of migraines. A doctor will attempt to explain all these things so you don't wind up doing things that you might regret deeply when something wrong happens to the baby. Because you'll be made aware of all the consequences and be held liable for each, you'll be better disciplined in avoiding things that may cause you to consume medication during the first few months of pregnancy, which may affect your child negatively.

In general, women who do not suffer in any other types of health problems other than migraines have a very low risk of harming their baby during conception. This is especially true if you don't experience regular migraine attacks. Consultation with a doctor before conception could also rule out degenerative brain conditions such as tumors, hemorrhage and meningitis. Because if any of those are determined as the cause of the headaches, then they would need to be treated first before pregnancy can be pursued.

Doctors often advises pregnant patients to seek alternative medication before the use of synthetic ones. Often, it is in the best interest of the patient to significantly cut down on the stress inducing things and activities in her life. Yes, very few would argue that stress is one of the most common triggers of migraine. That's why removing the stress out of your life is probably the first advice a person suffering from migraine would get from any health professional. There is of course a huge difference from being wanting to eliminate stress and actually doing it. Usually, it involves doing habit altering steps. Most could be compared to baby steps, but even with modest changes to your way of living the positive effects it will bring surprises everyone.

Another important thing concerning migraine sufferers and pregnancy, induced labor could trigger a migraine attack. Your doctor should be well aware of any conditions you may have. Without this knowledge, your doctor may agree to you being given certain hormones to induce labor. When delivery time arrives, you will be prone to having headaches together with the pain of labor, which will make your delivery even more painful.

WHAT EMPLOYEES COULD DO WHEN MIGRAINE ATTACKS

Although they feel almost alike, migraines are different from headaches. For one thing, a migraine is a disease. And like most diseases, workplaces from many countries have duties to ensure that the environment they are subjecting their employees to doesn't aggravate migraine. This is of course harder to implement because of the fact that not all migraines are the same. All sorts of different things could trigger different migraines, which further compounds the responsibility of employers to make sure that their employees are protected when at work.

Employees who suffer from migraines often fall into the stereotype that they are slackers. In a workplace filled with people who do not have enough knowledge of the disease, the perception of workers who suffer from migraine is that they are whiners. They are viewed differently because they are irked with the light most people do not have a problem with; they have to be sent home at times; as well as the trip to the company clinic. All these instances does not favor employees with migraines. Thus, they have to be protected by special rules and considerations much like other people who have certain disabilities.

Other than performing poorly in the job when migraine pain strikes, employees who suffer from migraine are also confounded by instances when they have to leave for home early, medical costs and sick leaves. With that said, it's no wonder that businesses are losing estimated billions of dollars each year. And of course people who suffer from migraines are also debilitated in their financial capacity unlike those who does not have the disease. Experts have even found out that the unemployment rate for people with migraines is strikingly high (10%-20%) compared with the average. Although we still have a long way to go, more and more businesses are welcoming migraine sufferers.

If you suffer from migraine and are about to start a new job, you must be open about your disease with your employer and colleagues. Let them know what to expect when your migraine attacks and what they can do to help. As for your employer, he deserves to have medical proof to back up your claim. Never tell them a cover up story because that will only make things worse. Telling them the truth about your disease is your best chance of helping them to understand your dilemma. Do not be ashamed and cover up your disease with stories that are not true because people can immediately tell. This will only make them think that you really are a slacker and may put your career in danger. As for businesses, they must do their best to accommodate employees with migraines.

MINIMIZE VISUAL AND AUDITORY DISTURBANCES

Workers with migraine often complains about environments where there are bright lights and high intensity displays around. These are in fact common triggers for their disease. There are plenty of research to backup this claim. Hence, your workplace should reduce direct sunlight, projectors and flashing lights from affecting employees with migraines.

Employers can setup partitions in place to block these distractions from affecting employees concerned with migraines. Make sure that the work floor also isn't bombarded with noise of high volume music as this might also cause migraine. Employers can also provide computer glare guards to any employees who request them. Full spectrum lighting installation is more suitable to all employees including those with migraine compared with regular fluorescent lighting.

Employers may also implement flexible scheduling so that employees with migraines and other disease aren't affected by their condition financially. If they leave for home early because of migraine attack, flexible scheduling ensures that they would be given the chance to cover lost productivity some other time. In extreme cases, employers should not rule out the possibility of allowing an employee with migraine to work from home. Employers should carry out regular maintenance of their company's ventilation and air conditioning.

As previously mentioned, businesses should have no discrimination against any individual suffering migraine or any other form of disease for that matter. To help with the employment process, here are some questions an employer should consider.

• What task would you assign to the employee?

• What task would he have trouble performing because of his disease?

• Will the employee have recurring issues of missing deadlines, productivity, and punctuality?

• How can you help resolve these problems?

To ensure that a business follows the existing requirements of workers with migraines approved by your government, here are further questions to consider.

• Is the physical layout of the work floor compliant with the government's requirements?

• What equipment do the employees with migraines commonly use?

• What is the kind of lighting and noise level that my employees with migraine will be comfortable in?

• How many visual and auditory distractions are present in our workplace?

Once these questions are answered, the next step is to find solutions for each of them. You'll want to look at altering the physical arrangement of the work floor to optimize it for people with migraine, this is especially valuable if there are more than a couple of people with the same headache concern. Secondly, you can introduce products that are available to specifically help employees with migraine perform much more efficiently at work.

RARE KINDS OF MIGRAINES

People with migraines do not all have the same kind of disease. Admittedly, there is a common form of migraine that most are afflicted with. However, there are rare varieties that you should be aware of.

Basilar Migraine

This form of migraine is more commonly known as basilar artery migraine. This is no doubt a very rare kind, which is potentially very harmful. In the early days, people believed that it only affects teenage girls and young women. Thanks to modern research though, we've seen that it can happen to both sexes. This type of migraine has terrible symptoms that include partial blindness, double vision, nausea, vertigo, continual vomiting, slurred talking, incoordination, lack of touch sensation (that could occur in only one or both sides of the body), debility, and general disarray. What makes matters worse is that this form of migraine could lead to stroke or TIA (transient ischemic attack).

Ocular Migraines

This is also sometimes called retinal migraine and is considered another rare form. It's known for repeated attacks that causes loss of vision in only one eye of the sufferer. The effect usually lasts for more than a few minutes but doesn't last more than an hour. This form of migraine is triggered mostly by bright lights that can lead to partial or complete blindness. Once the loss of vision goes away, the sick person is left with a severe headache that lingers in the entire head of the patient.

Hemiplegic Migraines

This character is acquired naturally from the genes of a person, but there are still more rare cases of sufferers who experience this even when no family member has had this in the past. Temporary paralysis is one of its prominent symptoms. Other symptoms include weakening of the lower portions of your body and more than an hour of headache. Hemiplegic migraines often advances early on in the childhood of the individual.

Ophthalmoplegic Migraines

This form of migraine puts stress and pain in the muscles that surrounds the eyes. It can also eventually lead to paralysis of those muscles. Symptoms include droopy eyelid, double vision, and visual disturbances. Ophthalmoplegic migraines are actually considered as a type of neuritis, because it leads to inflammation of the nerve. Consequently, some experts are even disputing if it should remain classified as a rare phase of migraine, which is plausible. Children are often diagnosed with this kind of migraine. The sad thing about this is that when it hits, it could last for long periods.

Status Migrainosus

Status Migrainosus causes pain and nausea that is so painful that patients often need to be hospitalized. This form of migraine could last for more than seventy two hours. A person suffering from Status Migrainosus is also in danger of being dehydrated. It is said to be caused by certain medications. When you have this form of migraine, it is best if you can get to an emergency room very quickly and then you can receive treatment consisting of pain killers and fluids.

Abdominal Migraines

This kind of migraine sets itself apart from other kinds of migraines because the pain the patient feels isn't isolated in the brain but also occurs in the abdomen. That's why the symptoms it causes include nausea and vomiting.

Migraines That Only Occur In Women

Some migraines are only afflicted on women because it has something to do with the hormone cycle. These migraines are often caused by the menstruation oscillations of women and oral contraceptives. Another cause is pre-menopausal and menopausal stage. Don't be surprised that these events in a woman's life can also lead to headaches.

The above are migraines that rarely occur and are not widespread. However, it is more important to note most of these migraines are associated with very high levels of pain. Therefore, it is very important that a physician has made ready a medication plan for you should the migraine occur anytime.

TEN MOST EFFECTIVE MIGRAINE CURES

The main problem that people have about treating migraine attacks is that there is no single cure that serves as a magic bullet for migraine treatment. There are different things that trigger migraine headaches, and trying to avoid all of them will be complicated and impossible. Fortunately, there are various cures that you may use in order to deal with the different symptoms of migraines. Here are ten of the most effective treatments that you may try out the next time that you experience this condition.

Cut Back on the Caffeine

Among the different kinds of food that trigger migraine, caffeine-rich foods and drinks stand out. Taking too much caffeine will lead to the worst headaches. Most of the time, migraine headaches are not the result of too much caffeine intake, but of caffeine withdrawal. In order for you to avoid headaches, cut back on the coffee and do so slowly and surely.

Skip the Aspartame

People who often complain about migraine often experience this condition due to their uninformed intake of a substance called Aspartame. Companies that use this substance to manufacture their products have gone great lengths in order to cover up the link between Aspartame and migraine. While moderate intake of Aspartame will do nothing to harm you and cause you headache, too much intake of this substance will lead to the worst headaches that you will experience in your life.

Stop Smoking

If you are a regular smoker, then there is a chance that you are also a frequent sufferer of migraine. In addition to the different health hazards that come with smoking, resisting the urge to light up just so you can avoid horrendous migraine headaches is added to the list. When you are experiencing a headache, see to it that you do everything that you can in order to avoid a situation that will expose you to smoke; even to secondhand smoke. This will not only keep your migraine from getting worse but will also make it easier for your body to battle the different symptoms of your condition.

Stop Taking the Pill

Women who take the contraceptive pills are more susceptible to experiencing migraine than the ones who do not. Contraceptive pills and their effects on the body's natural composition make migraines worse. You do not have to go entirely off of the pill just to control your migraine headaches. For some people, changing the brand of birth control pills that they use has done wonders. If changing brands does not work, then it may be time for you to look for other means of contraception that will not alter your body's natural hormone composition.

Dim the Lights

If you are experiencing a migraine headache, you can alleviate your condition buy dimming the lights and closing your eyes for a while. Bright lights trigger migraines and placing yourself in an area that has harsh lighting will do nothing for you. If you experience headaches regularly, then it will be a good choice for you to alter the lighting in your home permanently. Install softer and filmier bulbs. Go with lamps instead of harsh fluorescent lights. Try to take frequent breaks from working on your computer or install an anti-glare film on your monitor in order to keep your migraine attacks from getting worse.

Skip the Cheese, Wine, and Chocolate

If you are experiencing migraine headaches, then it will be a good idea for you to limit your intake of wine, chocolate, and cheese. Aged wine and cheese contain an amino acid known as tyramine and chocolates contain phenylethamine. Eating these substances and acids will not only trigger migraine headaches, but will actually make migraine attacks worse. If eating your share of these foods cannot be avoided, then make sure that you limit your intake of these food options.

Switch to Milder Scents

If you have a habit of splashing on cologne and perfume every morning, then you should consider switching to sweet-smelling body wash instead. Harsh odors and aromas may help you smell good throughout the day, but may also cause you to experience bad headaches. Switching to mild soaps, body wash and lotions will help you remain fresh throughout the day without making you prone to migraine headaches.

Get Moving

Getting active is a great way to battle the symptoms of migraine. Enrolling in an aerobic activity and attending classes regularly will improve your blood flow and cardiovascular activity, thus making you less susceptible to migraine attacks.

Stay Grounded

If you are a frequent traveler, choose to go by land instead of taking a flight to your destination. Taking these alternative means of transportation will limit your exposure to changing cabin pressure.

THINGS TO AVOID DOING DURING MIGRAINE ATTACKS

When it comes to dealing with migraine headaches, it is not enough that you undergo the necessary treatment. You should also avoid activities that will make your headache worse. Here are some of the things that you should avoid doing during migraine attacks.

Avoid Giving into your Cravings

For most people, food is the biggest trigger for migraine headaches. Actually, studies show that eating migraine-inducing foods is the main cause of severe migraine attacks. If you are experiencing extreme migraine headaches, make sure that you steer clear of foods that will make your condition worse. Skip foods that contain nitrate, like lunchmeats, cheese, chocolate, hotdogs and the like. If you are feeling hungry, stick to natural and healthy food that will nourish your body without subjecting it to a chemical overdose.

Avoid Caffeine

Caffeine and caffeine withdrawal are pretty high on the list of things that trigger migraine attacks. If you are used to ingesting much caffeine, then you should try to limit your consumption of this agent. However, you should avoid going cold turkey, because withdrawing from caffeine will not do you any good.

Avoid the Changing Climate

If you are suffering from a migraine attack, try to find a weatherproof area that will protect you from extreme changes in the weather. Fluctuations in the pressure and temperature will only make your condition worse. If you are traveling, put on the right type of clothes that will allow you to maintain constant body temperature.

Avoid the Cigarette

Smoke, whether inhaled directly or ingested secondhand, will trigger your migraine and will make headaches exponentially worse.

Avoid Too Much Visual Stimuli

Avoid changes in lighting that will trigger and exacerbate headaches. Take note of the condition that you subject your body to when you work on the computer or watch television. If you find that doing any of these things expose you to high levels of visual stimuli, then you should avoid these activities if you are experiencing a migraine attack.

Avoid Stress

While it is impossible to completely avoid stress every day of your life, you should do what you can in order to limit the stress levels that you experience regularly. Too much stress triggers migraines and immersing yourself in stressful situations during migraine attacks will only make you feel worse.

Avoid Overmedication

People often take painkillers in order to deal with migraine headaches. However, it is a common practice to increase the dosage of painkillers if the recommended dose fails to give you the result that you want. Instead of ramping up the dosage, try looking for an alternative treatment. Overmedicating will only lead to a condition called "rebound headache". If you find that taking pain killers have worked for you in the past yet you fail to experience the same result in the present, look for other brands and other treatment options that you may use in order to deal with the different symptoms of your migraine.

Avoid Ignoring Supplement Therapy

Believe it or not, a lot of vitamin supplements and herbal remedies have proven to be effective in treating headaches brought about by migraine. Avoid seeing these options as ineffective means of treatment and consider trying them out the next time that you experience a migraine attack.

Avoid Strenuous Activities

In case of a migraine headache, it will do you well to isolate yourself from areas that will stimulate you visually and aurally. Try to find a dark and quiet place that will serve your temporary refuge. Lay your head down, relax, breathe regularly, and try to fall asleep. You will feel better the moment that you wake up.

Avoid Skipping Personal Assessment

In order for you to feel better, you need to observe your body and find out what you can do to make yourself feel better despite your migraine. If you find that you have a high temperature, take a washcloth, wet it with cold water, and place it on your forehead. Use warm water if you are feeling cold. Balancing your body's temperature will help relieve your headache.

Avoid a Hectic Schedule

Enjoy a slow day every once in a while. While a slow routine may seem boring, enjoying your downtime will help you ease the different symptoms that come with a migraine attack. Make sure that you also enjoy regular sleeping patterns every night, in order to limit the possibility that you will experience frequent headaches.

Avoid a Sedentary Lifestyle

Exercising regularly will help you deal with migraine attacks. Achieving a physically fit body will make you less prone to suffering headaches and will make your body stronger and more able to deal with the symptoms of migraine.

Avoid Skipping Physician Appointments

Most of the time, people who suffer from frequent migraine keep their doctors in the dark despite regular headaches. Doing so will limit you from finding the different cures that will help you with your condition. As much as possible, tell your doctor or your physician about the pain and discomfort that you experience. This way, your doctor will be able to give you ample advice as to how to deal with your condition.

Consulting with your doctor will also help you find the best possible cure for your condition. Before taking any form of migraine medication, try to consult a physician and see whether that treatment option will give you the relief that you are after.

RECOMMENDED HOME REMEDIES FOR MIGRAINE

While migraines can't be considered a life-threatening condition, the effect of having an intense amount of pain suddenly striking your head can be a great hindrance to your everyday life. And while prescription medicines are available to help alleviate the pain, sometimes, the best cure for migraines can be found right at your home, or in your backyard.

Most of these remedies are readily available in your home, or you may be able to reproduce them very easily. If you're one of those people who frequently suffer from migraine attacks, then you may try these remedy methods.

Herbal Medicines

It's been proven through the years that different kinds of herbs are effective in treatment of certain diseases, thanks in part to the constant study dealing with the effectiveness and safety of different plants. Moreover, migraines are no exception.

One of the most popular herbs for migraine treatment is the Tanacetum parthenium, better known as Feverfew. This plant is usually grown in some households as a simple ornamental plant, and is one of the oldest known herbal treatment for migraine headaches, hence the name. This is made possible because feverfew plants contain parthenolide and tanetin, chemicals that helps control the expansion and contraction of the blood vessels in your head, which are the main reasons for migraine headaches. While feverfew supplements are readily available in the form of tablets and tincture forms, most physicians recommend consuming it while it's fresh, to ensure maximum effectiveness. This can easily be achieved by just picking out the leaves at your garden (if you have them cultivated), and serving them as toppings in your salad or sandwiches.

Lawsonia inermis, also known as the Henna plant, are proven to reduce the pains caused by migraine headaches. To make a quick headache remedy using Henna, simply dip a few henna flowers in vinegar, and rub them on your head whenever you suffer from a migraine attack.

Chamomile is also another effective migraine headache relief, in the same manner as Feverfew. A recommended treatment using it is to simply take a sip of chamomile tea whenever a migraine attack occurs, to help reduce the pain it incurs.

While not readily available at home, extracts from the Gingko Biloba plant has also proven to be helpful in curing migraine headaches. The recommended dosage for taking Gingko Biloba is 120 mg, which is already enough to help ease the pain.

As with any herbal treatment, before taking them, it's always advisable to consult a physician first, as some people might induce an allergic reaction to certain plants when taken.

Ice Packs & Cold Compress

Since migraine headache is caused by expanding blood vessels, cold temperature application can help in contracting the blood vessels in the head to return them to normal size. Therefore, applying either an ice pack or a cold compress in your head will help relax your head from the migraine pain. Just apply the pack at certain areas on your head, and alternating positions from time to time. Repeat this for three minutes until the pain subsides.

Proper Diet & Nutrition

As always, prevention is always better than the cure itself. A proper diet can also help in managing your migraine symptoms, preventing them completely.

The most essential nutrients for migraines are magnesium and niacin. Studies show that migraines can be due to low levels of magnesium in the body, which helps to relax the body. And to relieve migraine pains, a substantial level of niacin is needed by the body.

The best sources for niacin and magnesium are nuts and green, leafy vegetables. But some other fruits and vegetables, as well as fish, are good sources, too, especially when those fruits are taken in juice form.

THE BEST BOOKS ON MIGRAINES

Who told you that no one is reading books these days? Well, that is partly true. None of the physical books that you can touch and hold is flying off their shelves, but their digital counterparts are still raking in huge profits for digital eBook distributors like Amazon. If you plan to take part to some of this earning, then writing about migraines is a great way to start. Just imagine how many millions of people out there are afflicted with this disease, which brings with it an unimaginable amount of pain for the sufferer. That is why, each of those people who suffers from migraine doesn't mind at all spending for anything that could help them with their disease. A book that talks about how one can cure and relieve the symptoms that comes with migraine has a good chance of becoming a seller.

For people who are always on the lookout for the best resource, you still have to be mindful with your purchase though. Remember that not all books are created equal. You want to end up buying a book that will really help you cope up with your condition. Keep in mind that just about anyone savvy enough about the internet could submit a book and slap a good cover in there. Sadly, there are people victimized by these purchases that hardly contain anything helpful about migraines, which may even infuriate the buyer and trigger what he or she is trying to evade.

A good way of making sure of your purchase is to not skip due diligence. Fortunately, for you today, we've also done the effort to direct you to books that are more exhaustive about migraines. We've taken out all those useless resources you may end up buying if you're not too careful.

"What Your Doctor May Not Tell You About Migraines: The Breakthrough Program That Can Help End Your Pain" - by Alexander Mauskop

The strength of this book lies within its focus on natural therapy in relieving the symptoms brought by migraines. If you want to find out what are over-the-counter supplements that can lessen your spending with expensive drugs just to control your headaches, you'll find this book very useful.

"Breaking the Headache Cycle: A Proven Program for Treating and Preventing Recurring Headaches" - by Ian Livingstone and Donna Novak.

This book is written with a unique take based on the perspective of its author. This book is different from probably anything else you've read about migraines because its author is convinced that migraines are brought by a far bigger problem than we usually think of. The author points towards an overly sensitive nervous system, hence no regular medication can totally cure migraines. The author then introduces unique methodologies or what they call as "containment" programs to keep migraine from worsening. These methods include breathing exercises, diets, and becoming more social.

"All In My Head: An Epic Quest to Cure an Unrelenting, Totally Unreasonable, and Only Slightly Enlightening Headache" - by Paula Kamen.

If you want to read a book filled with a the thoughts of a first person who's also suffering the same amount pain as you, then this book is what you're looking for. In addition, the author tries to set this book apart because it touches mostly on alternative medicine that usually originated from the east. These things include yoga, acupuncture and even magnets. The book will also mention a patient's aura, and that migraine has a lot to do with a person's aura deviating from the norm.

"The Women's Migraine Survival Guide: The Most Complete, Up To Date Resource on the Causes of Your Migraine Pain and Treatments for Real Relief" - by Christina Peterson.

Since the majority of people suffering from migraine are women, it's important that we have an entire book dedicated to offering advice about migraines that occur in women. Most of its contents talk about menstruation, pregnancy, menopause and other migraine scenarios that can only be associated to women.

"The Headache Prevention Cookbook: Eating Right to Prevent Migraines and Other Headaches" -by David & Laura Marks

The whole idea of the book is that we are what we eat. The author suggests that the most natural way of fighting the harsh effects of migraine is to incorporate the diet systematic approach to your diet. The end goal of this book is for the reader to once and for all identify the type of foods that triggers his or her migraine so that he or she can totally avoid its consumption in the future.

"Conquering Your Migraine: The Essential Guide to Understanding and Treating Migraines for all Sufferers and Their Families" - by Seymour Diamond and Mary Franklin.

When a person suffers from migraine, depression almost always follows. This is what experts love about this book. It not only trains the patient on how to handle his or her disease, but it also tries to educate the closest people with the patient such as families and friends.

We Want Your Feedback on This Book!

Our main purpose is to make sure that our readers get value from the books we publish and that they have a good experience with all of our products. We are always working to improve our books and other products with every revision and update.

Every piece of feedback makes a difference in this process. And we would appreciate yours as well - whether it is good or bad.

Please take one minute to let us know what you thought by following this link:
http://checkmatemg.com/feedbackmigraines

www.ingramcontent.com/pod-product-compliance
Lightning Source LLC
Chambersburg PA
CBHW070826290526
45795CB00002B/851